WEIGHT LOSS FOR WOMEN OVER 30

7 NATURAL METHODS TO LOSE WEIGHT WITHOUT STRESS

Matt Ejik

CONTENTS

"The body achieves what the mind believes." - Not known

INTRODUCTION

It becomes more harmful the more weight you gain. If you don't do anything about it, illness—whether it takes the shape of diabetes or a heart condition—is guaranteed to manifest. Before reaching the point when you can no longer control your weight, you must be proactive in losing weight. It's not necessarily important to have a toned and sculpted body, but rather to be at a healthy weight. The abs can be worked on later; for now, you only need to lose a little additional body fat.

This eBook will help you lose the first 10 pounds, which is something we all find difficult. It's remarkable how small lifestyle adjustments, which center around a healthy diet and regular exercise, may help you drop 10 pounds.

CHAPTER ONE

BEGIN WITH WHAT YOU DRINK

The first step to weight loss is what you drink. People fail to recognize that the first step in shedding the initial 10 pounds is what they consume. In reality, most people are unaware that they may mistakenly believe they are hungry when they are truly dehydrated and thirsty. Water is also marvelous. Your body weight is made up entirely of water, over 66%. Water is essential for maintaining a healthy weight for the same reason.

Therefore, get lots of water. The suggested daily intake is eight glasses, although it can take you some time to get there. Your body needs a ton of water. Water not only removes all the poisons from your body, a retail establishment or food market that can handle precisely 8 water glasses. These are fantastic tools for losing weight since you can fill them up, freeze them, and then have fresh, cold water all day as the ice melts. You can also drink your water at room temperature if you don't mind. It just matters that you are obtaining the water that your body needs.

Drink a glass of clean, fresh water to start your day. Drink one as soon as you awaken in the morning. Your body won't have to struggle against dehydration, which will aid in its reactivation. In addition, after consuming a glass of water, you won't require such.

Before you start eating, sip some water. Drinking water will help you feel fuller naturally, reducing the amount of food you need to eat. Drink some water along with your meal. Drink something after every bite to help you feel filled without feeling bloated and to help you finish your meal more quickly.

Additionally, drinking water as you eat will hasten the digestion of your food, causing you to experience fullness more rapidly. Try to avoid soda as much as possible. All sodas are heavily sugar-sweetened. It's best to eliminate as much of your diet as you can.

Diet soda is still soda, too. Despite having less sugar, it still contains harmful chemicals and ingredients for your health. When consuming soda, follow it up with a glass of water. Keep in mind that caffeine also dehydrates you. Decaffeinated sodas still include small levels of caffeine and the same amount of sugar, making them not significantly healthier.

Don't believe what you hear about fruit juice being healthy. In actuality, juice contains a sizable amount of sugar. If you're in the mood for a glass of juice, opt for fresh fruit juice rather than juice with added flavors and colors. Making your own fruit juice is even preferable. Be careful not to add too much, though.

Furthermore, try to drink your tea and coffee black if you must have them. Black tea or coffee can be beneficial to your health as long as you drink plenty of water to balance the caffeine in them. Caffeine is also not beneficial for you because it alters activities in your body, such as your metabolism.

Another type of tea that you can drink freely is green tea. Over 4,000 years ago, green tea was utilized as medicinal in China. It supports the digestive system, can ease an excessively full stomach and has been connected to a lower chance of developing cancer.

In addition, it's better if you can avoid drinking alcohol. Although a glass of red wine does offer heart advantages, most alcoholic beverages are just fattening. Particularly fattening beer. Depending on the ingredients they include, cocktails can make you fat.

Take whiskey with Coke as an example. The Coke is undoubtedly fatty, but the whiskey might not be. Additionally, most people get the munchies after a few drinks, and when you're a little tipsy and hungry, you won't be able to make sane decisions about your diet. It's also common to overeat in the late evening, right before you pass out from a night of drinking. Simply put, the entire mix is poor.

Try dry wine if you must drink alcohol. Due to the higher sugar content in sweet wines, dry wine is preferable. Although dry wines do contain sugar, the majority of it has been fermented into alcohol, making them healthier for weight gain.

One more thing about coffee—not that it's always bad, but it's more intriguing than anything. Some claim that they shed more weight when they drank black coffee before working out.

Nutritionists speculate that it might be brought on by the body being pushed to use fat as fuel, however, there is no scientific evidence to support this. Hey, if you can handle black coffee, it's worth a go. Just keep in mind to stay hydrated while working out!

CHAPTER TWO

PROPER EATING

Okay, most people think of dieting when they think of losing weight and eating. Unfortunately, all of the available fad diets tend to cause people to gain weight. Why? Because they starve them to death, and the person eventually succumbs to hunger and eats everything in sight.

They also deprive them of their favorite foods. This is neither a way to lose weight nor a way to live. You are only causing yourself stress, which causes you to gain weight. So, when it comes to eating right, there are a few tips you can follow every day that will not deprive you of the foods you love but will treat those foods as luxury items, allowing you to enjoy them even more.

Consume fresh, water-rich fruits and vegetables. Tomatoes, watermelons, cantaloupe, kiwi, grapes, and so on are examples. All of those fresh and flavorful juicy fruits and veggies are good for you. These items contain about 90 to

95% water, so you can eat a lot of these and they will fill you up without adding on the pounds.

Eat fresh fruit instead of processed fruit. Anything that is processed has more sugar. Fresh fruits contain more fiber than processed or canned fruits. Increase your fiber consumption as much as possible. This usually entails consuming more fruits and vegetables.

When it comes to losing weight, vegetables are your best friend. There are numerous options available here, and you may want to try some that you haven't tried before.

The leafy green varieties are the best, and you should always incorporate them into a salad when possible. Salads are high in nutrients as long as you don't overdress them and pile on too much cheese. The leafy greens are also high in natural water.

Make informed food choices. Don't eat for the sake of eating. Animals eat instinctively, whereas humans eat only when their bodies require it. Don't eat on the spur of the moment.

Keep track of everything you eat, from the food itself to what you top it with. Because they are typically high in fat, garnishes and condiments can derail a healthy meal.

Master your sweet tooth. This does not preclude you from enjoying sweets; just don't eat them as a meal. Always keep in mind that these treats end up adding to an area where you don't want them to. Don't deprive yourself either though, because then you'll eat twice as many as you should.

Set and stick to mealtimes. Try to schedule your meals and eat them at those times. An eating pattern will assist you in controlling what and when you eat. Also, having 5 small meals a day is preferable to just one or two large meals. Simply eating once a day causes your body to feel starved, causing it to store fat rather than use it as fuel.

Also, don't eat until you're starving. This only causes you to overeat until you're full. Only eat when you are hungry.

Drink a glass of water first to determine whether you are truly hungry or not.

It's common for people to eat when they see food. They simply want to consume it; it does not imply that they are hungry. If you're not truly hungry, don't accept any food that is offered to you. If you feel obligated to eat it out of politeness, simply nibble; skip a meal.

Try to avoid snacking in between meals, but if you must, make sure it's a healthy snack. Try to find healthy snacks rather than junk food if you travel frequently.

Vegetables make excellent snacks. If you are experiencing hunger pangs, they can help you get through them. Because they are nutrient-rich and satiate hunger, carrots are wonderful.

By the end of the week, burn off the excess calories. Make sure to visit the gym or go for a longer walk if you feel like you have indulged excessively this week to burn off those additional calories. Avoid eating anything that has been fried. It is preferable to bake anything breaded. Foods that are fried are covered in fat and oil. Even after the extra oil has been removed, oil is still absorbed into the food item. Don't skip meals.

A minimum of three meals each day are recommended, but five small meals are preferred. This will prevent you from being ravenous during the day and overeating as a result. Fresh vegetables are preferable to canned ones, much like fruits. If you can eat your vegetables raw, that is even better.

The nutrients are lost when you cook them. If you must cook them, try to boil them just long enough to keep some of their crispness. Don't dunk them in butter either. It would be best if you could purchase organic vegetables free of pesticides.

Limit your egg consumption to one per day. The best option is to limit your egg consumption to three per week. Treat chocolates like a luxury goods. Purchase the best, and consume them infrequently. Each bite will taste even better if you take the time to appreciate it.

This will increase your enjoyment of the meal. Include foods from each food group in your daily diet. This is a fantastic technique to make sure you are getting all the nutrients your body needs and it aids in preventing any dietary deficits.

Additionally, avoid eating the same things repeatedly. Try new things to avoid getting bored with your current diet. Try to have to breakfast an hour after waking up. The greatest method to give your body the boost it needs is to do this. Avoid waiting till you are genuinely hungry. Although breakfast is crucial, you shouldn't overeat. The idea is that you're breaking the fast from not eating all night.

All food groups, including carbs, should be present in your diet. Your diet should consist of 50–55 percent carbohydrates. A significant source of energy is carbs. Diets that forbid carbs are harmful to you and just increase your cravings for them. You shouldn't lack any nutrients due to your diet.

Only 25–30% of your diet should be made up of proteins. The idea that meat should be the focal point of your meal is overemphasized. In reality, it is more appropriate to classify it as a side dish as opposed to the main meal.

Between 15% and 20% of your meal should be fats. This is all the fat your body needs. You'll be eating a lot of this in the diet in the form of cream, sugar, and other things. Eat more white meat than red meat (Chicken, fish, and some other poultry are examples of white flesh), Beef and pork are examples of red meat.

Try to eat as many vegetarian meals as you can. Even if you can't entirely cut out meat, this is still a better way of living. The better is to consume as many fruits and vegetables as you can. The more meat you eliminate from your diet, the more fat you may eliminate as well. However, protein is crucial, so be sure your choice enables you to maintain healthy protein levels.

White bread is good, but multigrain with high fiber levels is considerably superior. These breads provide a good amount of protein and are an additional app increasing increase your diet's fiber intake.

Eating pork in no way promotes weight loss. You will do better when trying to lose weight if you consume less pork. Bacon, ham, and sausage are among the foods made from pork, which has a high-fat content.

Try to cut back on your sugar intake. If you must sweeten your coffee and tea, look for an artificial sweetener whose flavor you enjoy. However, these activities should also be restricted because they are not particularly healthy either.

Attempt to graze five to six times daily. These are the snacks that we previously spoke about. Some people find that they lose weight more successfully when they never feel hungry, and you can achieve this by grazing on healthy foods.

Additionally, it keeps your metabolism active, which naturally burns fat. Don't worry about cheating, but avoid doing so during meals. Consume treats and your favorite cheat food solely for flavor. Share a dessert with the entire family if you desire one after dinner. You won't gain any weight, just the flavor.

Watch your consumption of fat. A gram of fat contains 9 calories. You can calculate the quantity of fat in those things if you know your overall calorie intake. Use less salt overall and make an effort to reduce it in half. One of the biggest contributors to obesity is salt.

CHAPTER THREE

COOKING TO LOSE WEIGHT

Here are some suggestions to assist you to lose your first ten pounds by simply altering your diet preparation. How food is prepared affects its nutritional value just as much.

Try baking those items rather than deep-frying them in lard or oil. When you bake, your food is not submerged in the butter and oil that frying submerges it in while it cooks. Use the non-stick cooking spray in place of oil. Additionally, non-stick pans require little to no oil at all.

Rather than cooking veggies, boil them. You may also steam them, which is likely the best way to consume foods like carrots, broccoli, cauliflower, and cabbage. Avoid foods with no or low-fat content. These food products are widely available, although they are not particularly healthful. Many of these foods are sweetened with a chemical or carbohydrate to improve their flavor.

These substances and carbohydrates are nevertheless converted by the body into sugar, which implies that fat is still formed from them.

Avoid being a diet crash victim. These are detrimental to your health and ultimately cause more harm than good. Usually, you will drop a few pounds in the short term, but as soon as you stop, everything returns, making your weight worse than before.

You ultimately reach a point where you must stop following a crash diet because you cannot thrive on one.

Whether it's liquid meals, desserts, or ice cream, chew it at least 8 to 12 times. Saliva is added to the food, aiding in the sugar's digestion. When you simply swallow food instead of chewing it, you flood your stomach with undigestible food.

Use high-quality extra virgin olive oil when cooking. It is more expensive than vegetable oil, but because of the superior health advantages, the price is justified. Olive oil helps to increase the elasticity of the arterial walls, which lowers the risk of heart attack and stroke. It has also been linked to a lower risk of coronary heart disease.

CHAPTER FOUR

MOVE YOUR BODY (EXERCISE)

There are two things you must do to lose weight, and one of them—eating healthy foods and drinking enough pure water—has already been described in great detail here. Get your body moving as the other thing you need to accomplish.

Exercise doesn't require you to buy a gym membership. In truth, there are several daily activities you may engage in to help your body start losing weight, as well as several workouts you can perform alone to accomplish so.

Don't give up if you don't start seeing results right away from working out, whether it's at home or in a gym. Getting your body in shape and starting to see results for longer than a week. When exercising, many people make the error of thinking that it takes too long and is ineffective.

When you initially begin working out, injuries might occur if you push your body too far. You are exerting pressure on your bones, joints, and ligaments when they are not ready for it. Do not assume that if you work out consistently for a few weeks, you will lose money; sadly, this is not how the body functions. The race is won by caution and consistency.

When you first start working out, weigh yourself, but don't use it as a gauge for how much weight you are shedding. Throughout the day, your weight changes. You might just end up giving up if you weigh yourself every day.

The fit of your garments is the best indicator of weight loss. You'll know that eating right and exercising help you if you start to feel like you're floating around in your clothes. Moving where you normally fasten your belt—tighter is better—is another sign that you're losing weight.

Reward yourself when you frequently check your weight and the way your clothes fit. Purchase a new pair of pants or a new pair of running shoes for yourself. As you work toward your weight loss objectives, this will support you in staying motivated.

Take a day off from working out to give your body a chance to recover. Every week, your body requires a day off. You can maintain your weight with three days of 30 minutes of exercise, but to start losing weight, you need at least four days of 30 minutes of activity, and five days a week is even better.

Gather knowledge on exercises and simple tasks you may complete at home. There is a ton of in-depth research on exercise accessible, and you may choose what will help you the most to achieve your weight loss objectives.

Browse the web or obtain some books on fitness and health from your neighborhood library or bookshop to learn more and how to burn off the desired number of calories you are trying to burn each week.

Try to find a workout partner. This person should share your commitment to exercise and weight loss. Finding a devoted relationship has several benefits, one of which is having someone to feel accountable to. It is simpler to get out of bed and go for a workout with someone when you know they are waiting for you. You wouldn't want to make your workout partner stand up, would you?

Take a rest when your body signals that it has had enough. You will begin to feel messages from your body once you have exercised for a while. When you are just beginning your fitness regimen, this is especially crucial when you're first starting your exercise regimen.

Gradually lengthen your workouts if you chose to do so. The same is true of your workout intensity. Pick a workout plan that works for your lifestyle. Everyone has a distinct lifestyle and works in a different field.

There is no specific time that you must or must not exercise. If you find that working out late before bed is calming for you, then do it. It's also fantastic if you prefer to exercise first thing in the morning because it helps you wake up.

Some individuals enjoy working out during their lunch hour to unwind from the pressures of their jobs or since they can only use that period. Move around instead of remaining still.

Do it if you can move around. Pacers benefit greatly from their frequent movement since it helps them stay healthy. You can think better through pacing.

The couch and the TV are detrimental to losing weight. Avoid sitting on it if you tend to become a couch potato. To reduce the amount of time you spend in front of the television, if necessary, place a less comfortable chair in front of it. In the case of computer junkies, the same holds.

Some individuals find their chairs to be more comfortable in front of their computers than in front of their televisions. (Of course, if you don't work from home and must spend hours at a time sitting in front of a computer, your chair is crucial.)

If your job requires you to sit all day, get up and stretch about every 30 minutes. The majority of today's occupations demand you to sit down in front of a computer. Make it a point to move occasionally if you have a job like this. Walking around while on the phone is essential If the chat is lengthy, you'll get a nice workout.

Use the stairs rather than the escalator or elevator. Despite being wonderful conveniences, these things make us exceedingly lazy. Additionally, taking the stairs can be quicker than waiting for an elevator to open.

Give up smoking. Although smoking may not directly affect your weight, it does cause unpredictable eating patterns and increases caffeine dependence. While running is one way to obtain your daily 10 minutes of cardio, there are other ways as well.

Try 15 minutes of brisk walking to stay in shape if you are unable to run due to a physical condition. If you have the time, you can walk almost any place. Consider walking or riding a bike if going to work or the store is close by. Even if it could take longer, you still get in a workout.

Keep the remote control out of sight. When trying to lose weight, remote controls are also bad. Without a remote, you might not even turn on the television, leading you to look for more engaging activities. If you don't have a remote, stand up and switch the station, or take a stroll instead of watching TV.

Bring in your catches. You should walk and fetch everything you need from the kitchen, the TV channel, the driveway, or the mailbox. It will benefit you greatly if you increase your daily walking.

Just take the stairs, or accompany it by walking or using the escalator. In between commercials, move around or perform easy workouts like crunches or bending over and touching your toes. Make every effort to increase your body's movement and blood circulation.

Play some music, and start moving. It goes without saying that the more you move, the better you'll feel and the more weight you'll shed. If you're on the bus or train, get off a few blocks before your stop and continue walking from there. This is a convenient method to get in a walk before and after work or en route to somewhere else.

Gyrate your pelvis to tone your midsection. These are obviously not exercises you would perform in public, but they are a fantastic first step in getting your body ready for more challenging stomach crunches. It keeps you loose rather than tight and is also helpful for your back muscles. When you walk, breathe through your nose. Maintain a normal gait while making an effort to tuck your stomach in. Soon, you'll start to feel those muscles tense.

EASY WALL PILATE WORKOUTS FOR A TRANSFORMED MIND AND BODY

Wall Core Strengthening

"The body achieves what the mind believes." - Not known

1. Investigating Wall Sit-Ups and Leg Raises

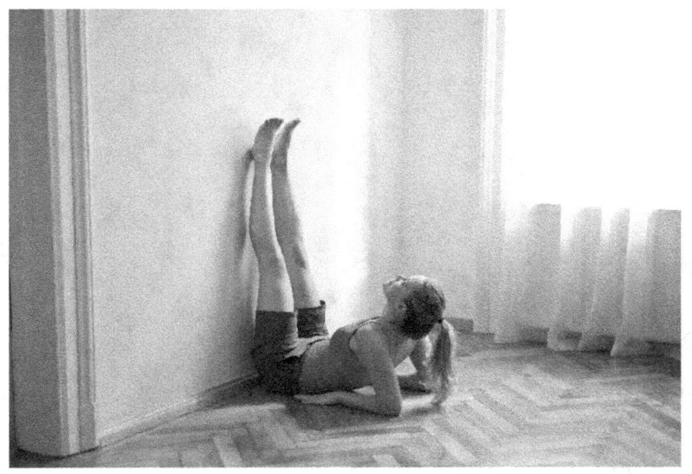

Wall Sit-Ups

Begin by reclining on the mat with your legs stretched against the wall. Lift your torso slowly towards your knees while engaging your core. Lower yourself back down with control. Aim for 10-15 repetitions.

Lie on your back with your legs against the wall. Lift your legs up and straighten them. Lower them without letting them hit the floor. Perform 10-12 repetitions.

2. Wall Supported Plank Variations

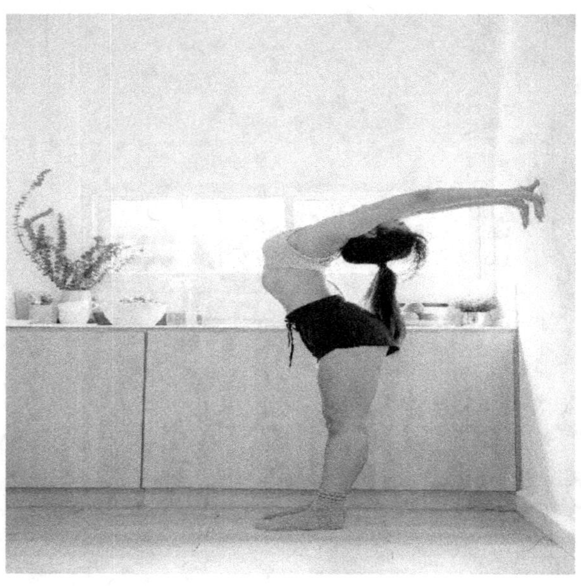

Wall Plank

Get into a plank posture with your forearms on the floor and your feet against the wall. Hold for 30 to 60 seconds, focusing on activating the core muscles.

Side Wall Planks

Create a side plank posture by resting one forearm against the wall. Maintain a straight line from head to feet by lifting your hips off the ground. Hold each side for 20-30 seconds.

1. Waist and oblique Strengthening Side Planks

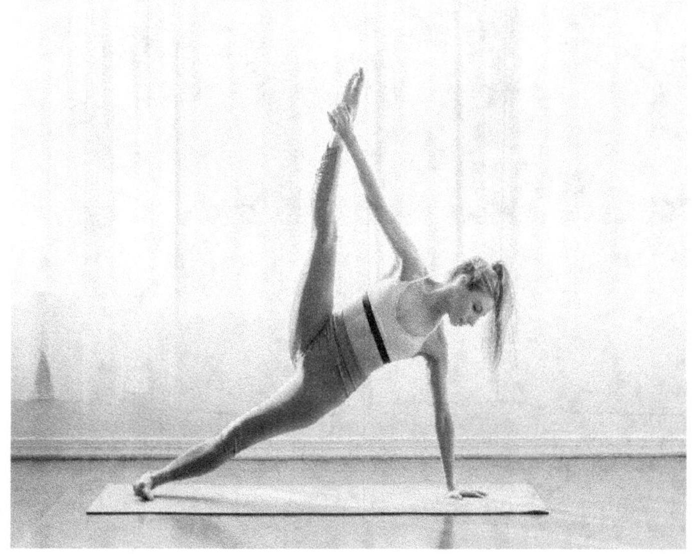

Wall Side Crunches

Stand with one shoulder against the wall, sideways. Raise your arm overhead. Crunch sideways slowly, bringing the elbow to the hip. Complete 12-15 repetitions on each side.

4. Pelvic tilts and abdominal engagement exercises are introduced.

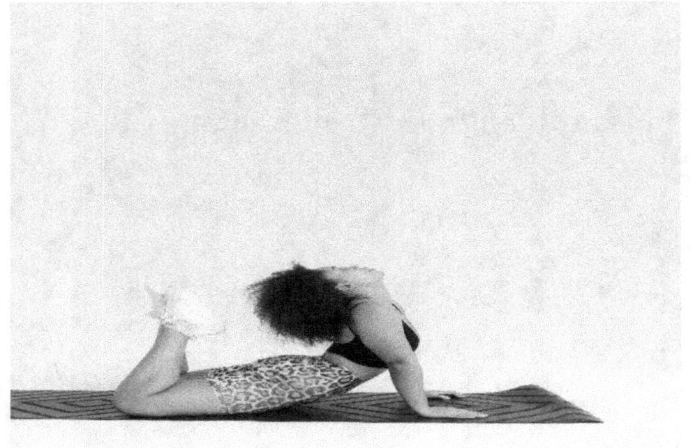

Pelvic Tilts

Lie down on your back with your knees bent and your feet against a wall. Tilt your pelvis forward and press your lower back against the mat. Hold for a few seconds before releasing. Repeat 10-12 times more.

Abdominal Engagement

Position yourself with your back to the wall. Pull your belly button towards your spine to engage your core. Hold for 20-30 seconds while breathing normally.

Conclusion

These exercises focus the core muscles, assisting in strengthening and toning while using a wall for support. Individual fitness levels may be used to vary the repetitions and length of each exercise.

1. Wall Stretches for Leg Flexibility

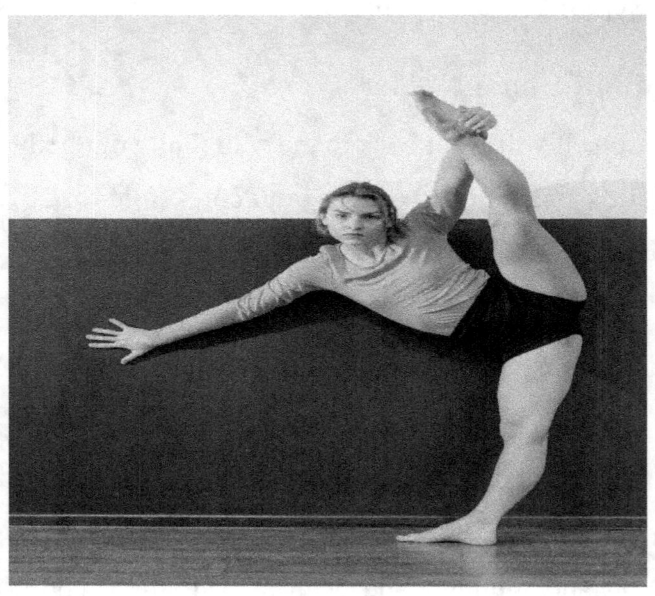

Lie on your back with one leg stretched up the wall and the other relaxed on the floor for a hamstring stretch. Pull the outstretched leg towards you gently, feeling a stretch down the back of the leg. Hold for 30 seconds before switching sides.

Quad Stretch

Face the wall and grab on for support. Bend one leg and bring your foot up to your glutes. Hold the foot with your hand until you feel a stretch at the front of your thigh. Hold each leg for 20-30 seconds.

2. Wall Supported Standing Balance Exercises

Single-Leg Balance

Stand near a wall and place a hand on it for support. Lift one foot off the ground while remaining balanced on the other. Hold for 20-30 seconds before alternating legs. Increase the length gradually as your balance improves.

Tree Pose Variation

Begin by standing near a wall. Place the sole of one foot on the opposing leg's inner thigh or calf. Find your center of gravity and hold for 20-30 seconds per side.

Increase Flexibility Through Wall Stretches

Wall Pigeon Pose

Lie back against a wall and cross one ankle over the opposing knee. Slide your foot up the wall, feeling the hip and glutes stretch. Hold for 30 seconds before switching sides.

Wall Cobra Stretch

Face the wall and lay your hands at shoulder height on it. Step back and forth, bringing your chest closer to the wall. Feel the stretch in your shoulders and chest. Hold the position for 20-30 seconds.

Including Yoga-Inspired Wall Poses

Wall Supported Downward Dog

Face the wall and lay your hands at hip height on it. Allow your body to bend forward, forming an inverted V shape as you walk backward. Feel the hamstrings and shoulders stretch. Hold the position for 30 seconds.

Wall Squats and Variations for Lower Body Toning

Wall Squats

Stand with your back against the wall and lower your body into a seated position, as if sitting in an invisible chair. Hold for 20-30 seconds or longer, focusing on engaging the thighs and glutes. Gradually increase hold time as strength improves.

Pulse Squats

Perform wall squats with a slight variation by pulsing up and down in the seated position. Aim for 10-15 pulses per set.

Targeting Glutes and Hamstrings with Wall Lunges

Reverse Wall Lunges

Stand facing away from the wall, hands resting against it for balance. Step back with one leg into a lunge position, bending both knees. Return to the starting position and switch legs. Perform 10-12 reps per leg.

Wall-Supported Forward Lunges

Stand facing the wall with hands placed on it for support. Step forward into a lunge position, keeping the front knee aligned with the ankle. Return to the starting position and alternate legs. Aim for 10-12 reps per leg.

Calf Raises and Leg Extensions Using the Wall

Wall Calf Raises

Stand facing the wall and place your hands lightly on it for balance. Lift your heels off the ground, rising onto your toes. Lower back down and repeat for 15-20 repetitions.

Wall Leg Extensions

Lie on your back with legs extended upward against the wall. Lower one leg down towards the floor, keeping it straight, then lift it back up. Alternate legs and perform 12-15 reps per leg.

Cooling Down with Lower Body Stretches

Wall Supported Quad Stretch

Stand facing the wall and grab one foot, bringing it towards your glutes. Maintain balance by keeping the supporting leg slightly bent. Hold for 20-30 seconds per leg.

Wall Butterfly Stretch: Sit facing the wall with the soles of your feet together. Gently press your knees toward the wall, feeling a stretch in your inner thighs. Hold for 30 seconds while breathing deeply.

Wall Push-Ups and Modifications for Upper Body Strength

Wall Push-Ups

Stand facing the wall, arms extended, and hands placed shoulder-width apart. Lower your chest toward the wall by bending your elbows, then push back up. Aim for 12-15 repetitions.

Incline Push-Ups

Place your hands on the wall wider than shoulder-width apart and perform push-ups. This variation targets different areas of the chest and arms. Aim for 10-12 reps.

Triceps Dips and Arm Exercises Utilizing the Wall

Wall Triceps Dips

Sit on the floor with your back against the wall, palms on the floor behind you, fingers facing towards your body. Lift your hips off the ground, bending your elbows to lower your body, then straighten your arms to return to the starting position. Aim for 10-12 reps.

Wall Arm Circles: Stand facing the wall with arms extended sideways. Make small circles in a forward direction for 20-30 seconds, then reverse the circles for another 20-30 seconds.

Shoulder Stabilization Exercises Against the Wall

Wall Shoulder Taps

Assume a plank position facing the wall. Lift one hand and touch the opposite shoulder, alternating sides. Aim for 10-12 taps on each shoulder.

Wall Y Raises

Stand with your back against the wall, arms extended straight out in a Y shape. Slowly raise your arms up, keeping them straight, and then lower them back down. Aim for 12-15 reps.

Incorporating Resistance Bands for Added Intensity

Wall Band Pull-Aparts

Secure a resistance band around a wall fixture or doorknob at chest height. Hold the band with both hands and pull it apart, bringing your hands towards your chest. Return to the starting position and repeat for 12-15 reps.

THANK YOU FOR READING

Thank you for reading this book, I believe you have acquired relevant insight to help transform your body to perfect fitness. Remember, Consistency in practicing the insights in this book is required to achieve maximum result.

A pleasant review and rating on Amazon will be highly appreciated.